Special Like Colin

Donna Nolte

AuthorHouse™
1663 Liberty Drive
Bloomington, IN 47403
www.authorhouse.com
Phone: 1-800-839-8640

First published by AuthorHouse 4/25/2011

ISBN: 978-1-4567-3108-3 (sc)

Library of Congress Control Number: 2011901421

Printed in the United States of America

This book is printed on acid-free paper.

authorHOUSE®

Colin is special. He can't run as fast as the other kids but he is the best cheering section ever. This makes his team happy.

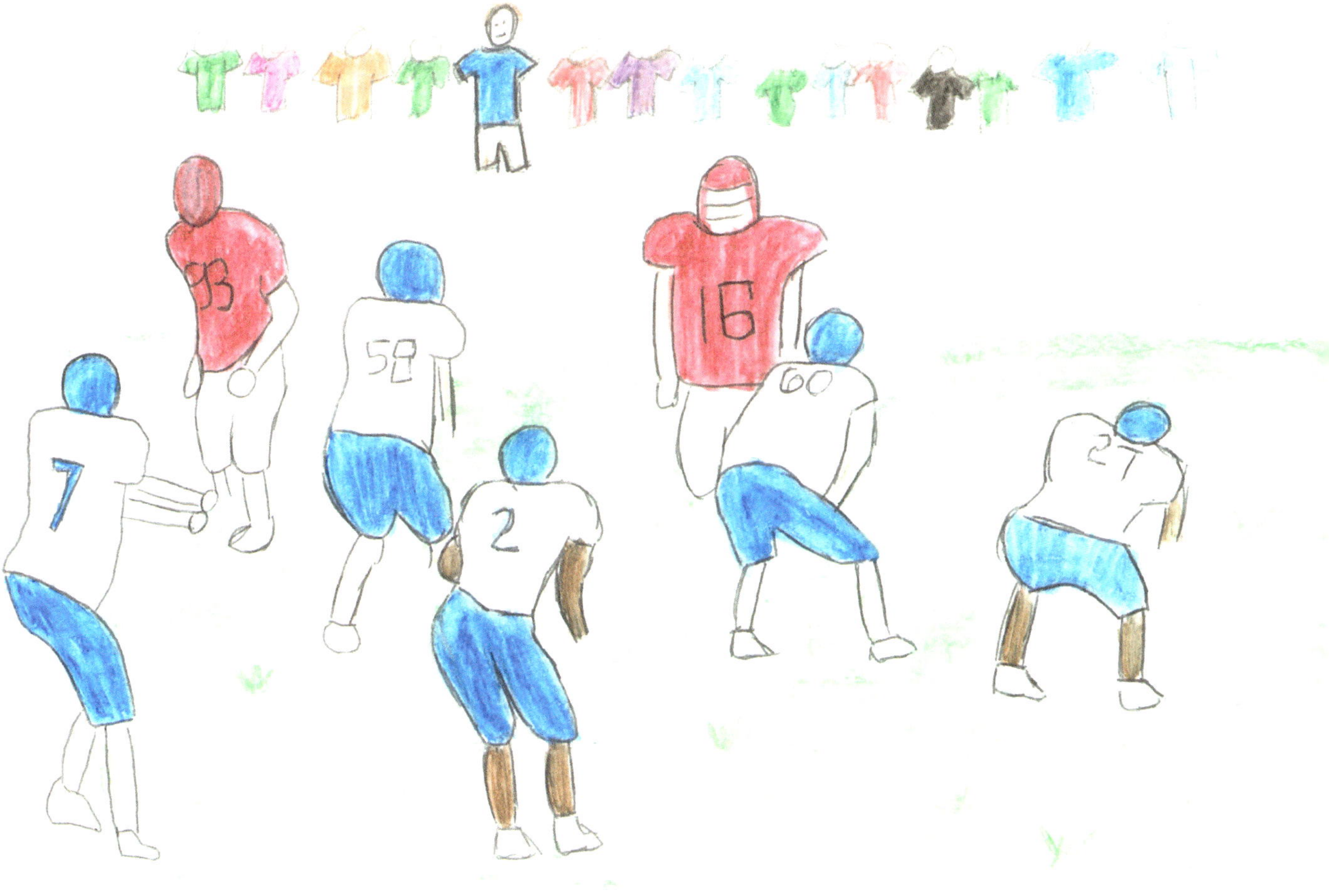
93
58
16
60
7
2
27

Colin can't play baseball as well as the other boys in his class but he can hit golf balls into the swimming pool. Every time. This makes his friends laugh.

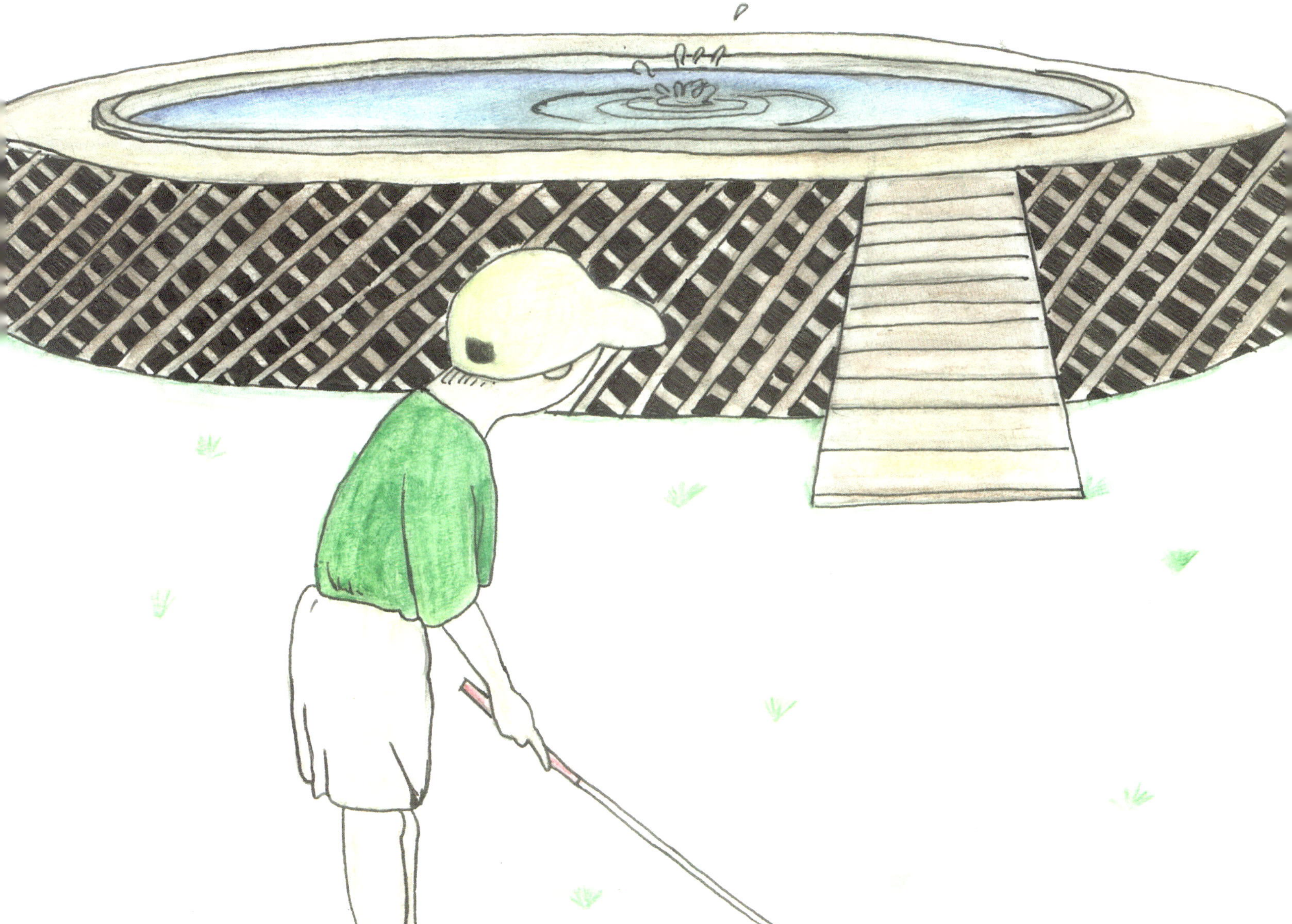

Colin can't do long math problems but he can play really hard video games and program the DVD player. This makes his friends happy.

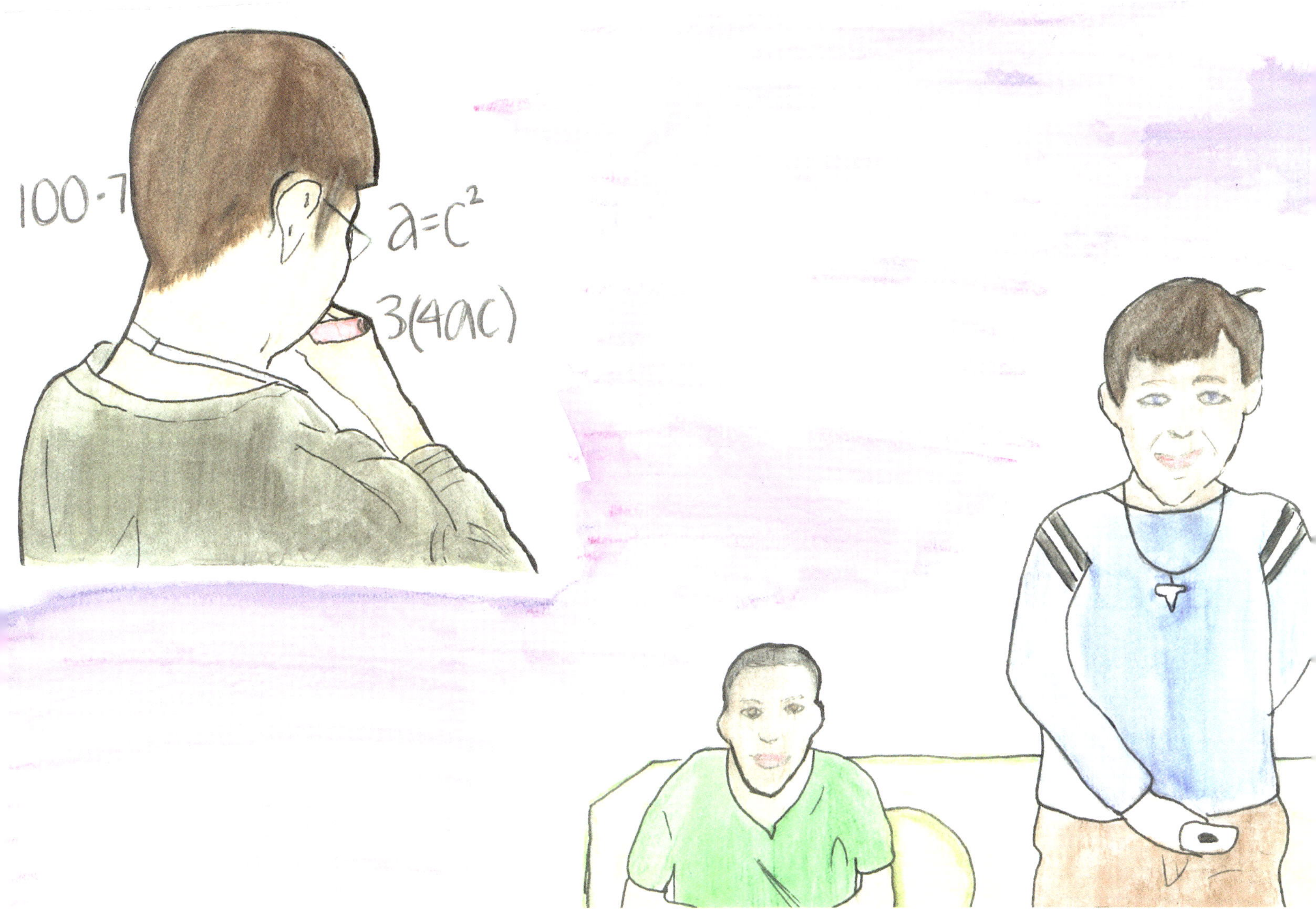
100-7
a=c²
3(4ac)

Colin isn't quite as quick on the football field as the others on his team but he celebrates the most when he scores and is the best dressed. This makes his friends celebrate, too.

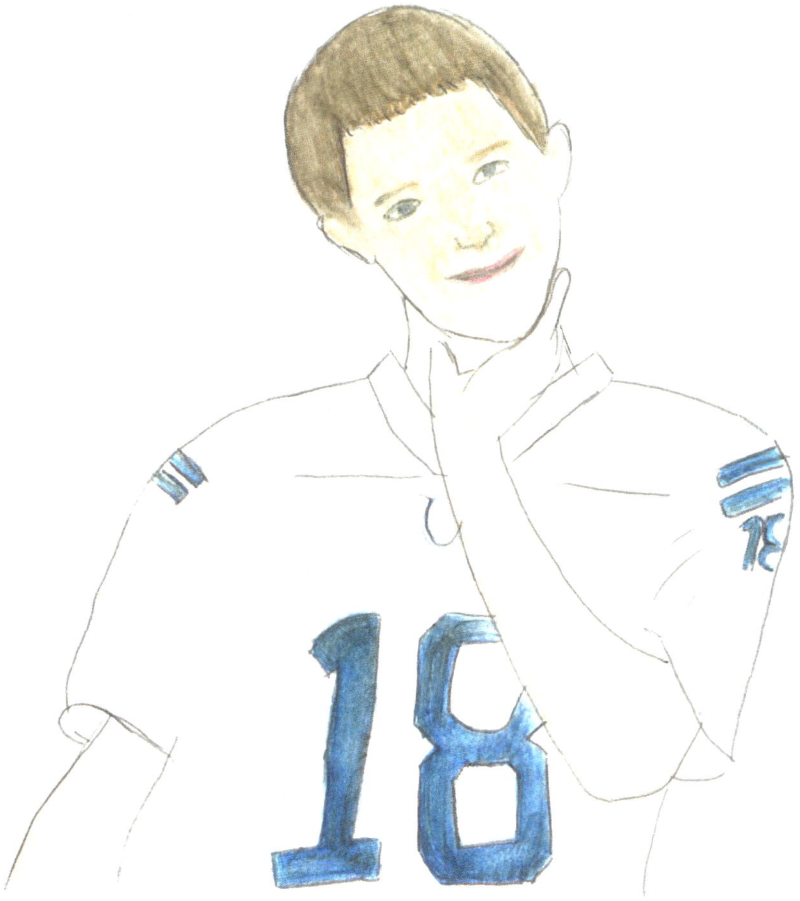

Colin doesn't understand all the rules of basketball but he can make a basket from a LONG way. This makes his Aunt Elisha a little jealous.

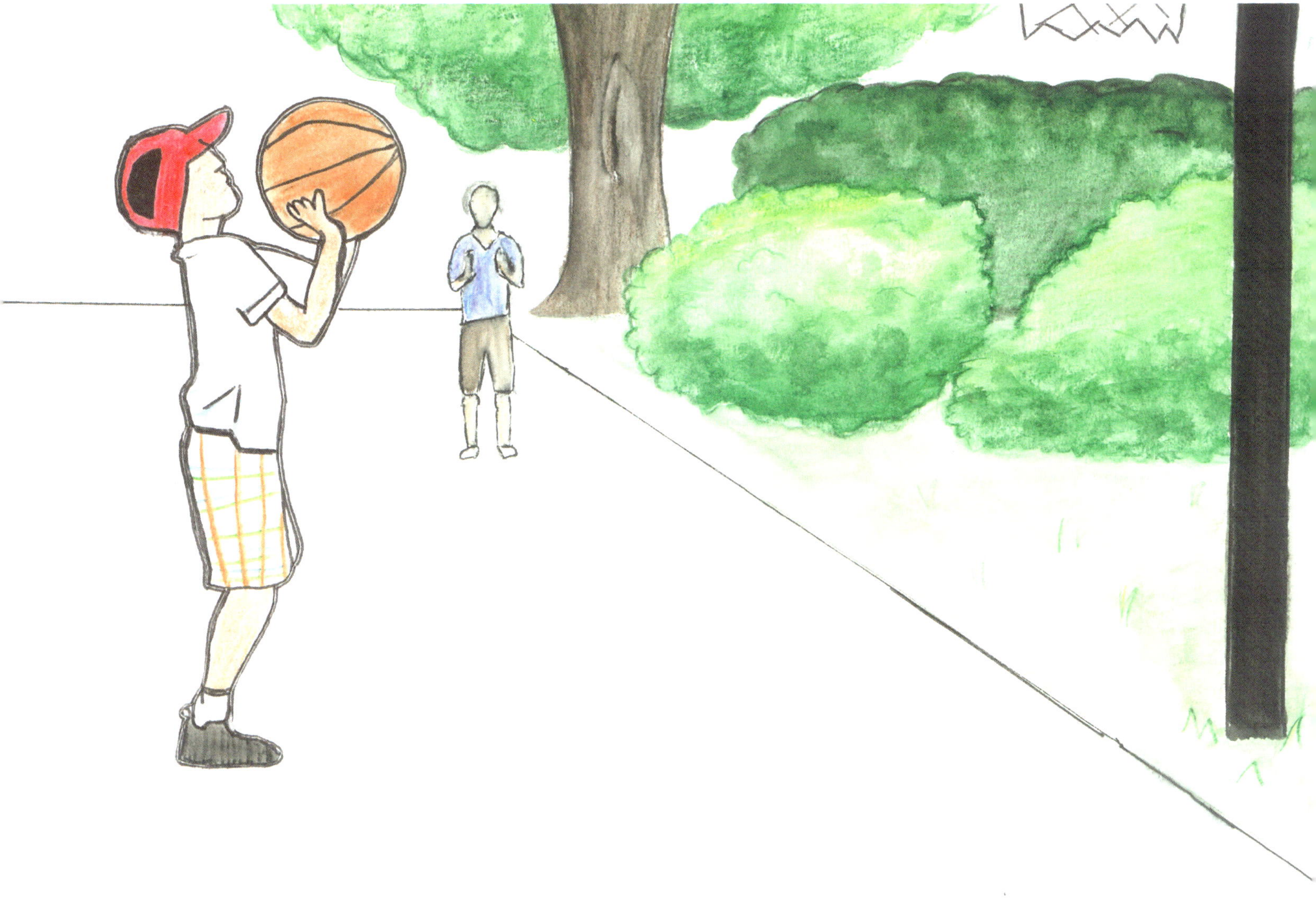

Colin takes lots of pictures. He can't always delete the blurry ones but most of them aren't blurry anyway. This makes his sisters laugh.

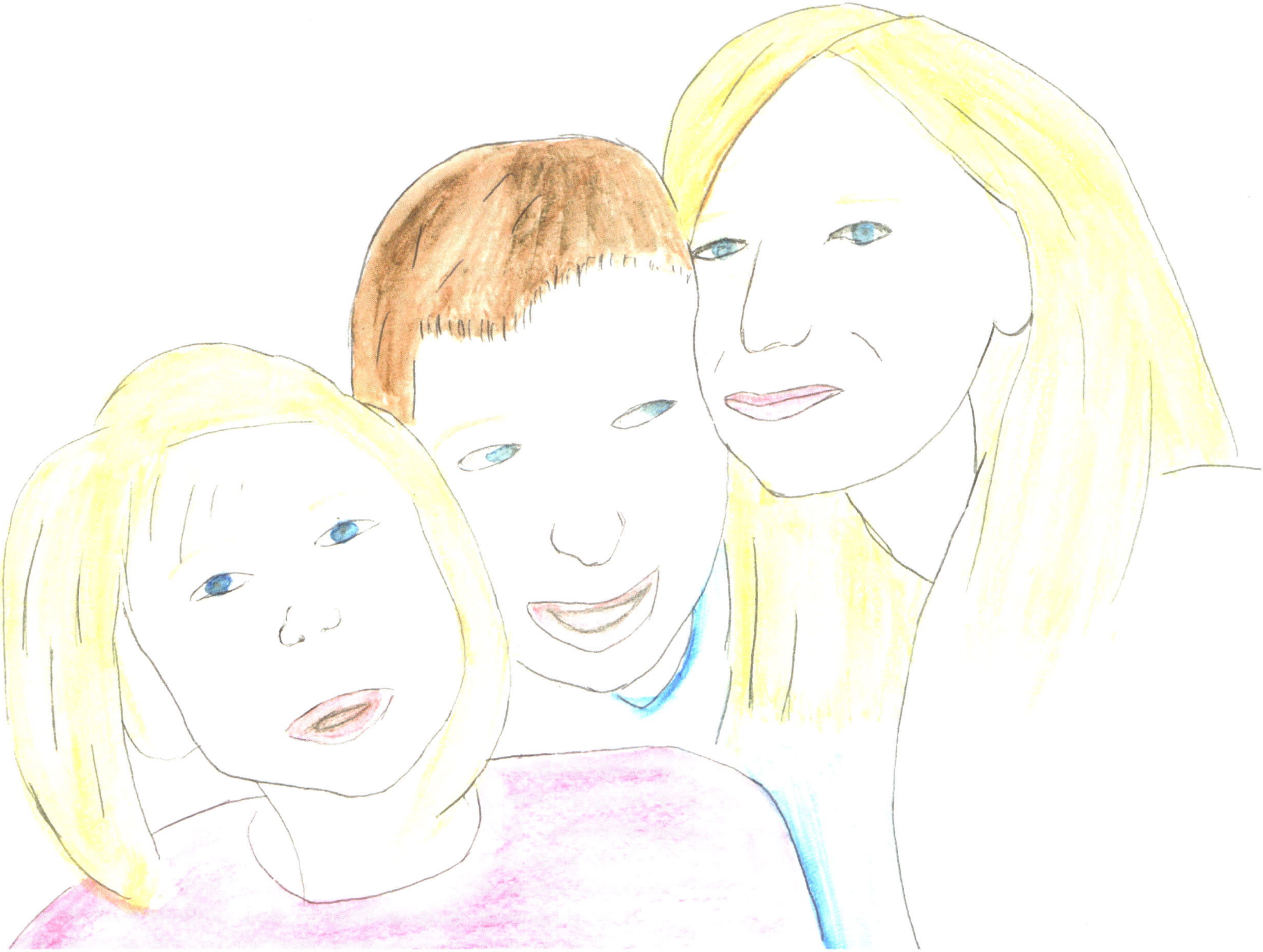

Colin doesn't always understand exactly what Father Thack is talking about but he knows the prayers by heart. This makes his church family happy.

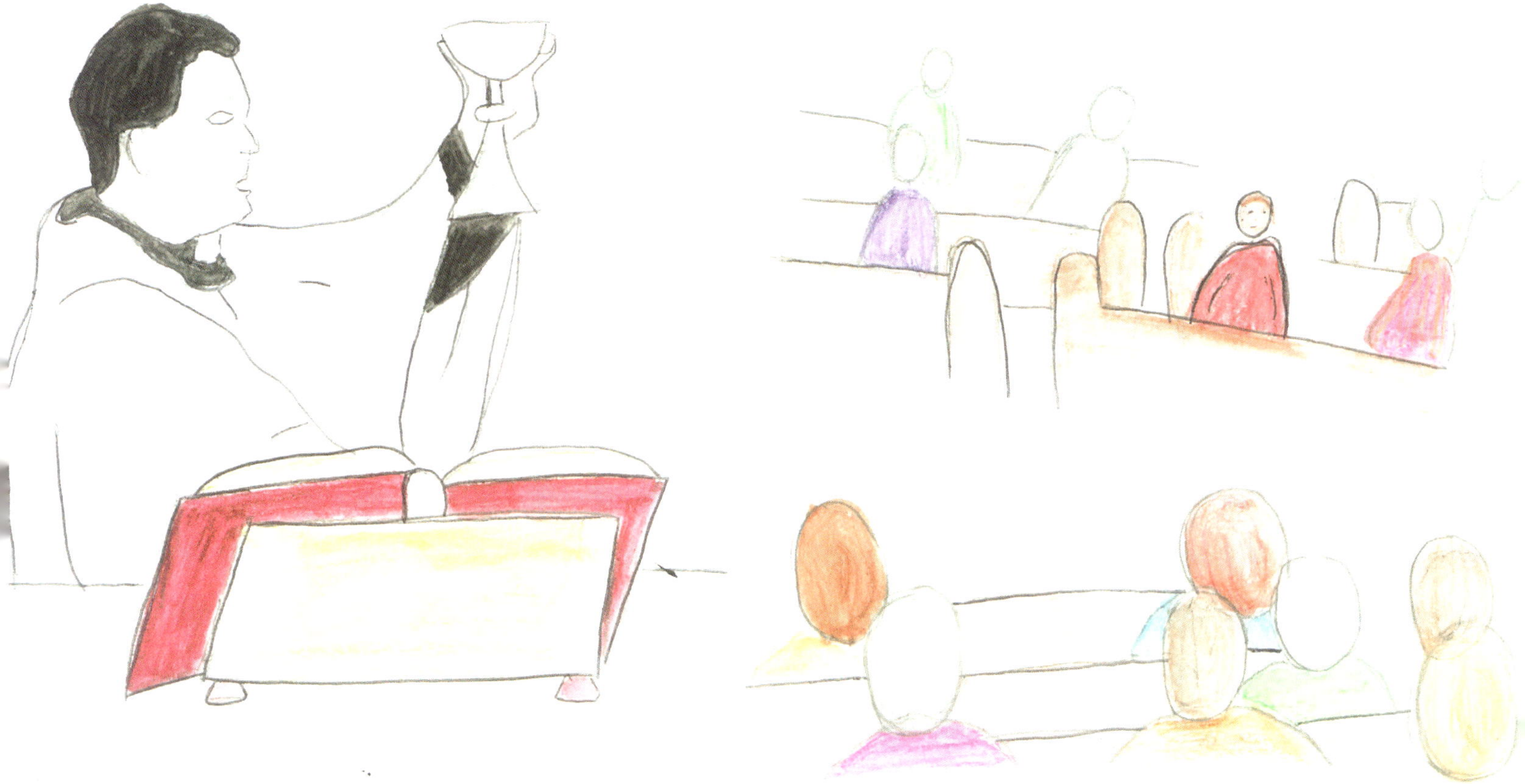

Colin might not be able to say the big words but his sister loves for him to read to her. This makes his sister smile.

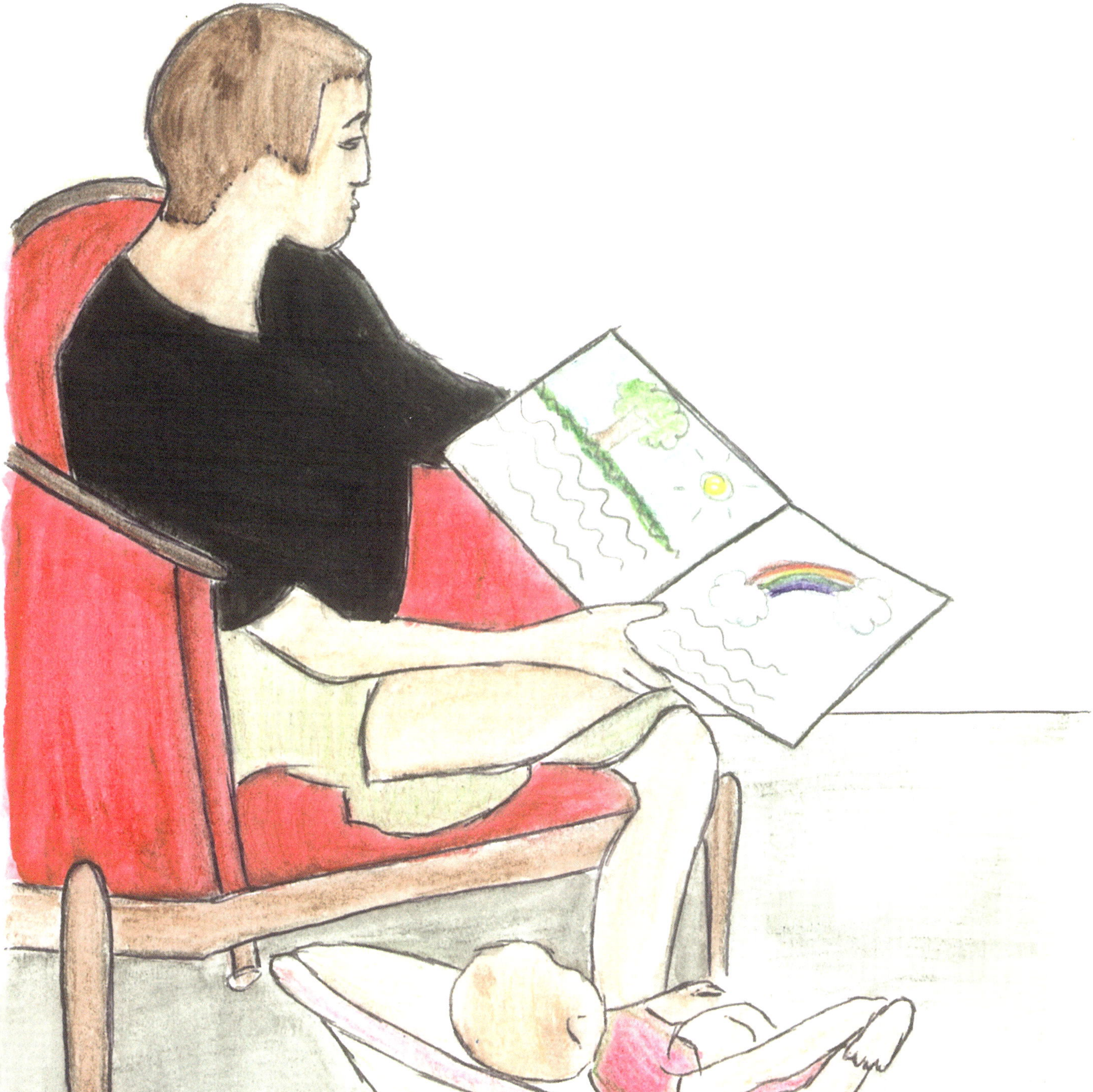

Colin doesn't always paddle as fast as others but he never turns the kayak over. This makes his Dad proud.

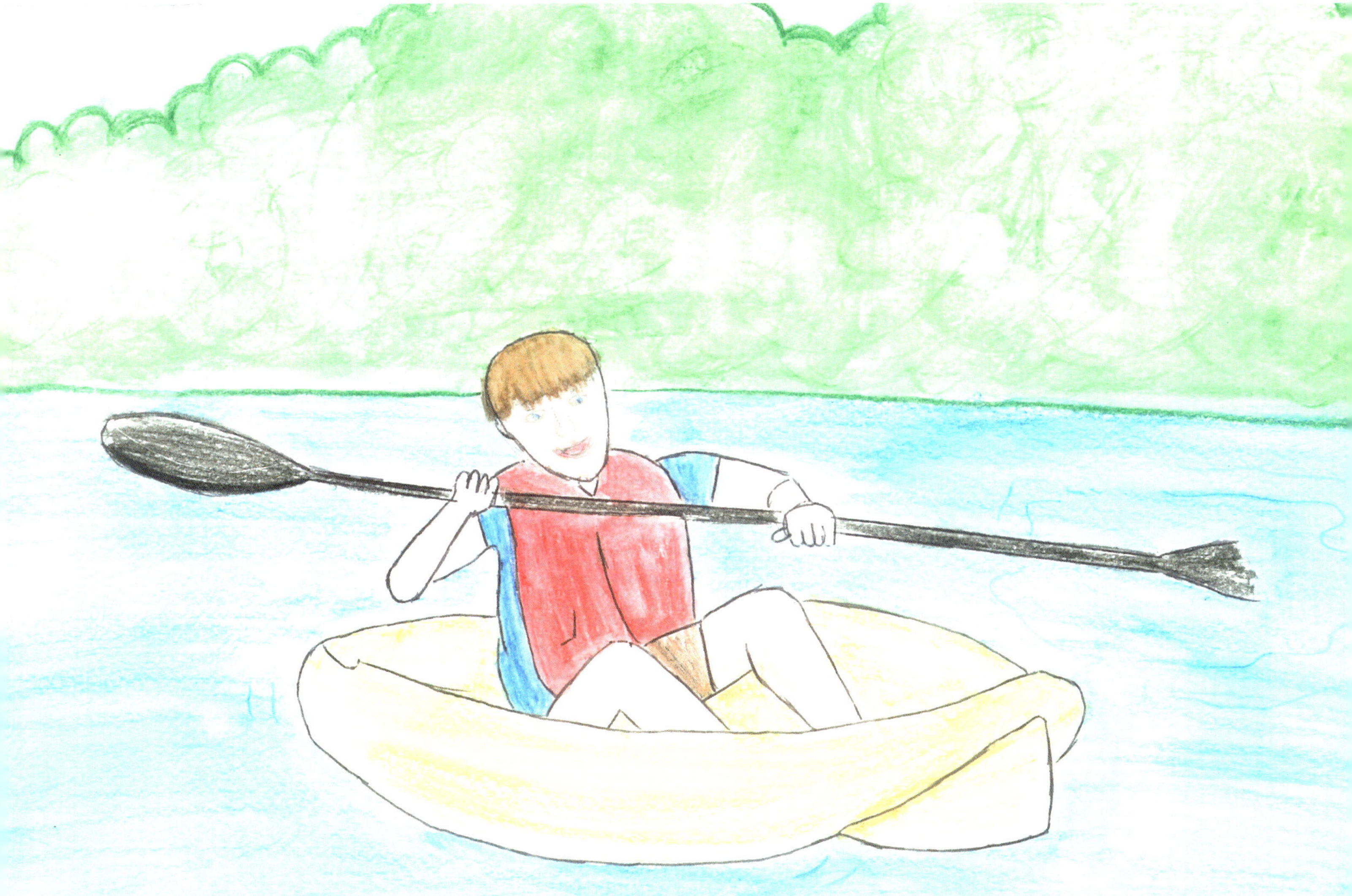

Colin is a skateboarder. He doesn't try the really hard skateboard tricks but he rarely ever falls.

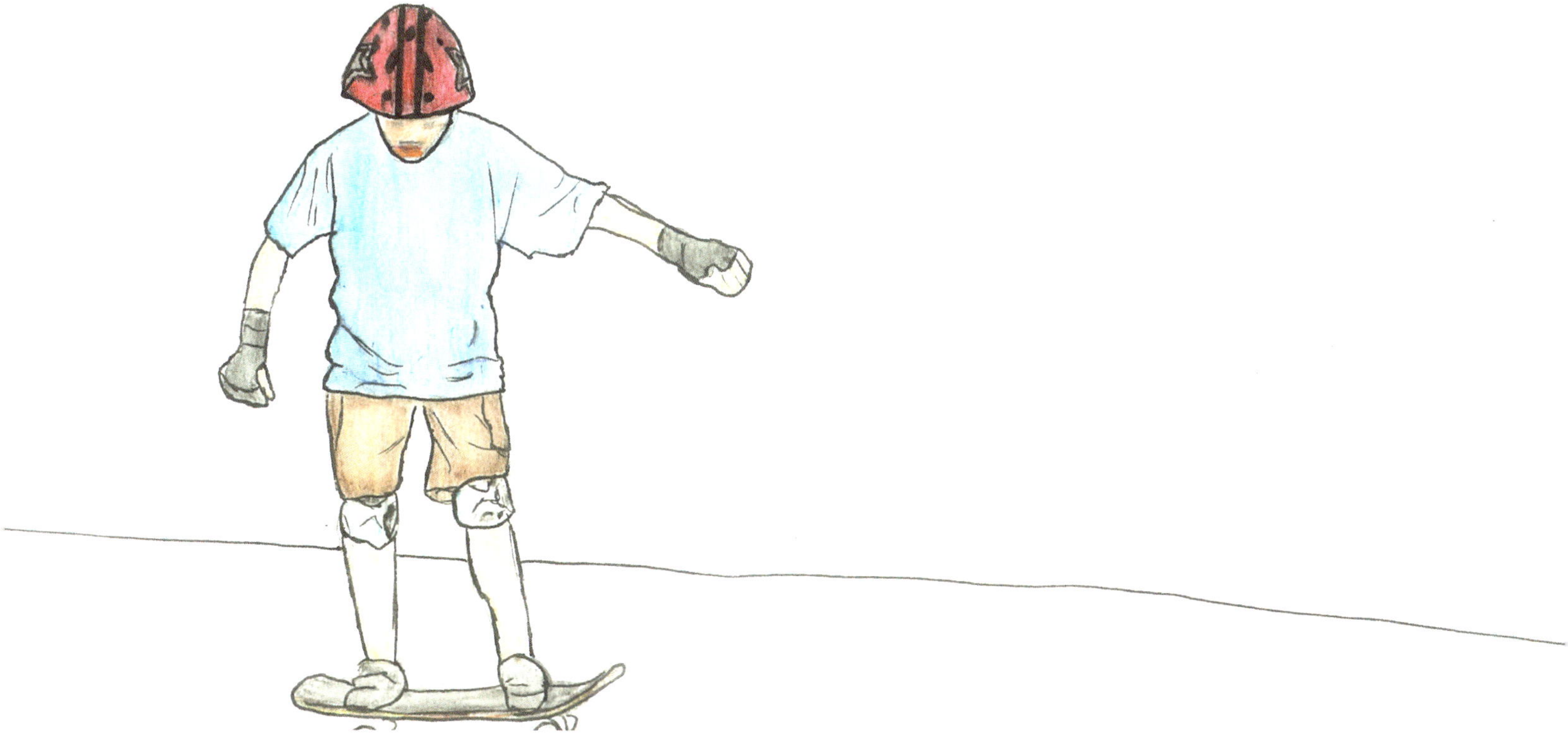

Colin doesn't always remember to pick up his clothes but he remembers everyone's name. This makes EVERYONE smile.

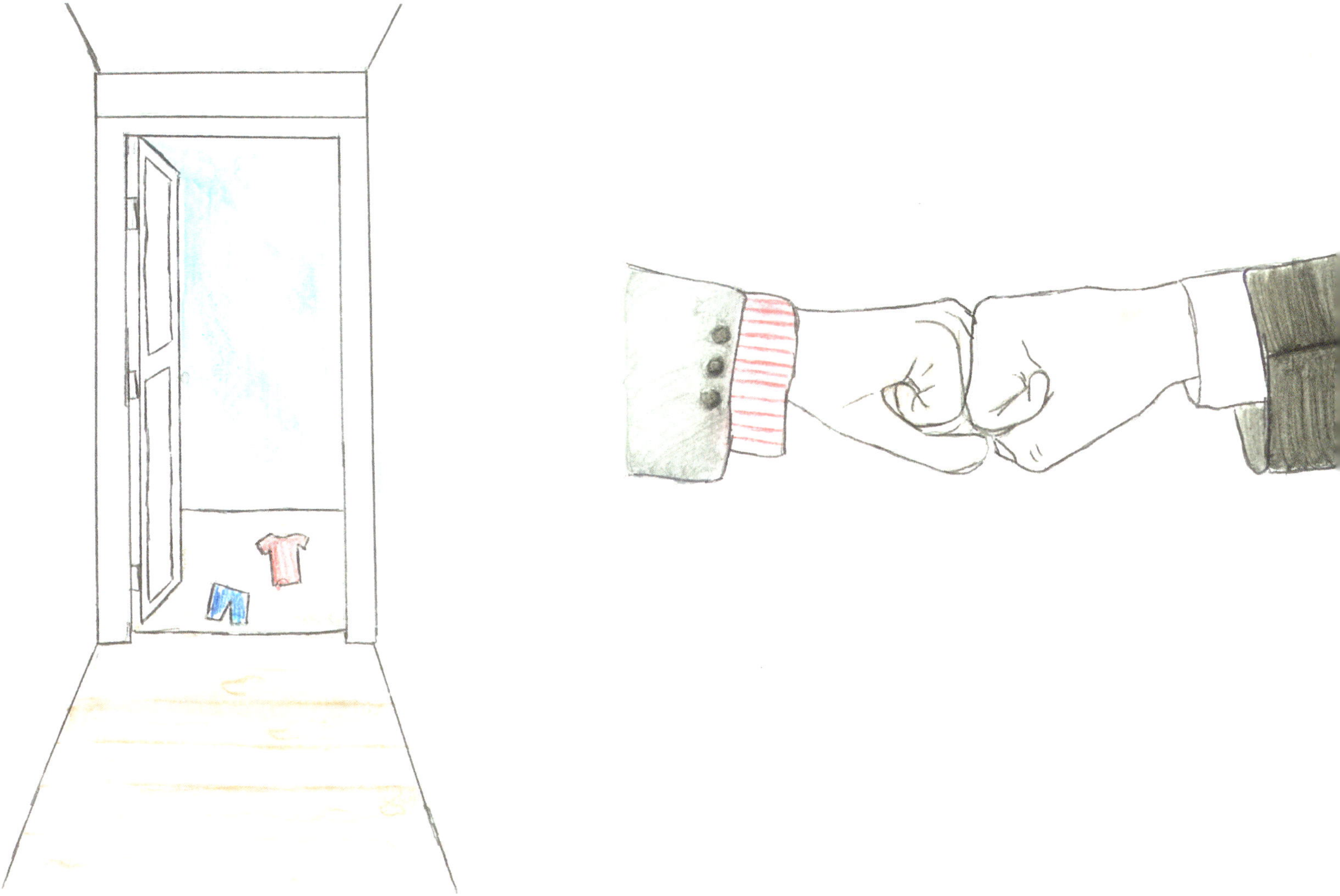

Colin doesn't always understand what the penalty is for but he always cheers for the Colts.

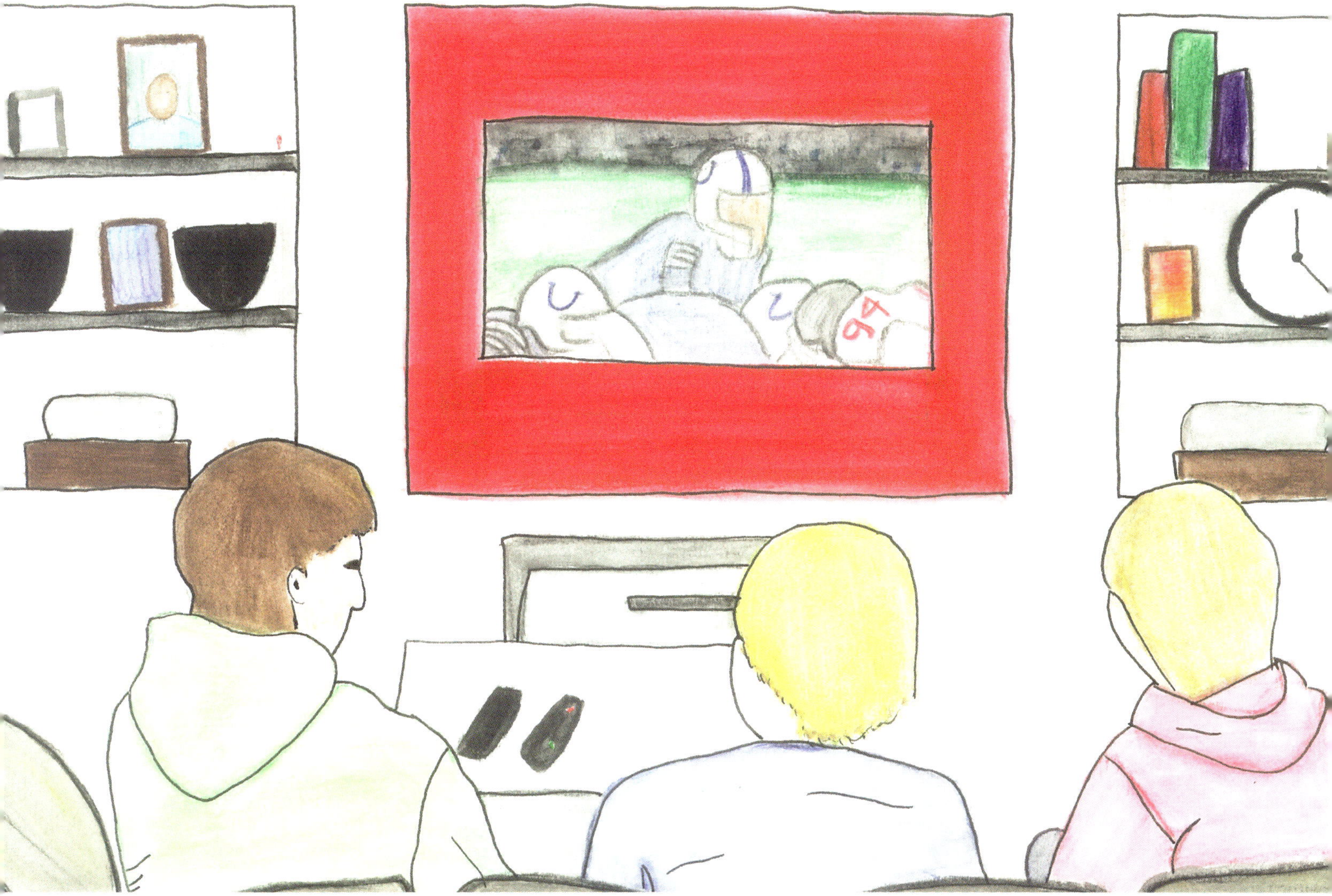

There is nothing that Colin can't do on a computer...

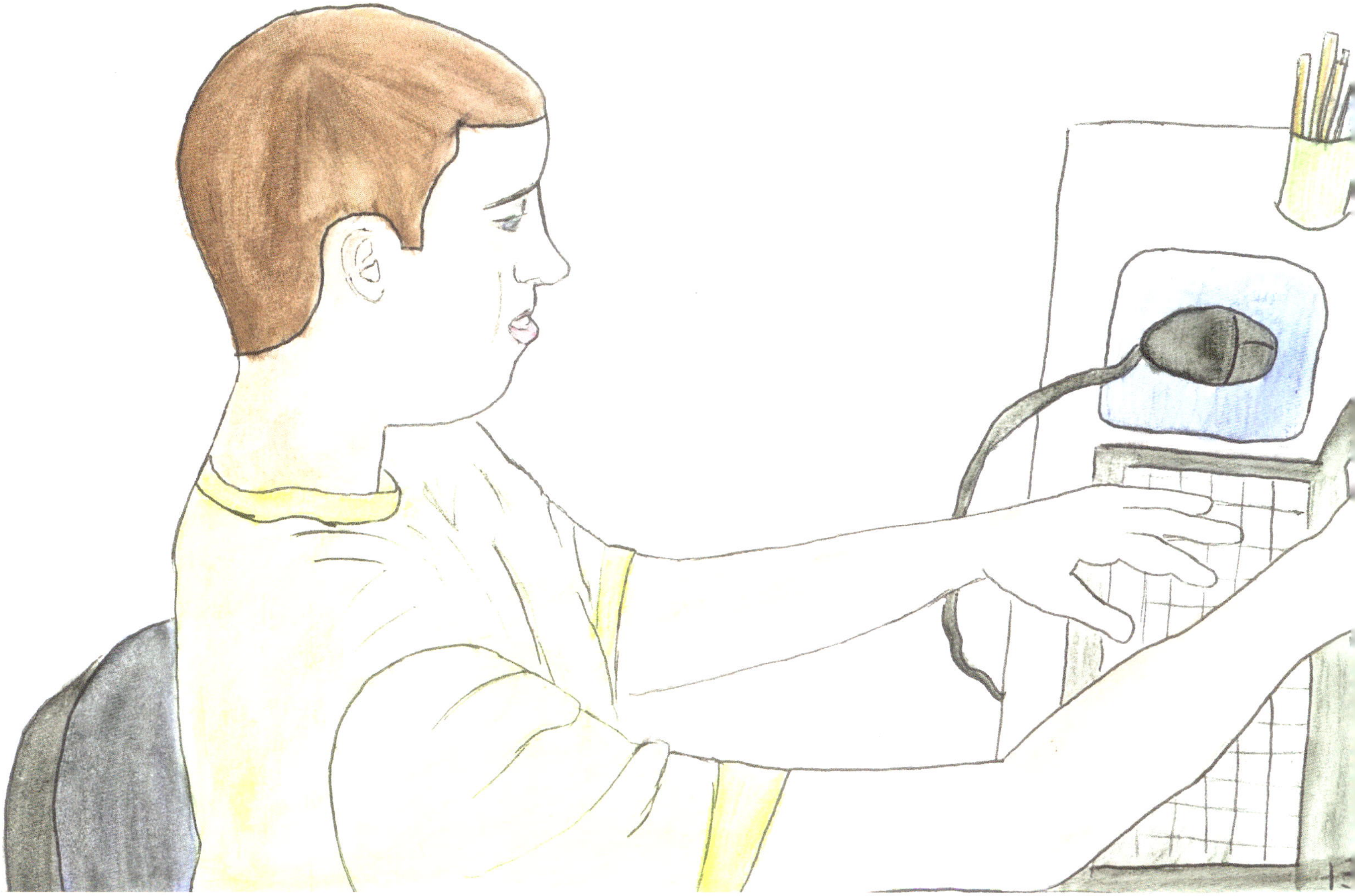

Colin doesn't worry that he runs a little slower. He's proud to be in the race. And that makes Colin a winner.

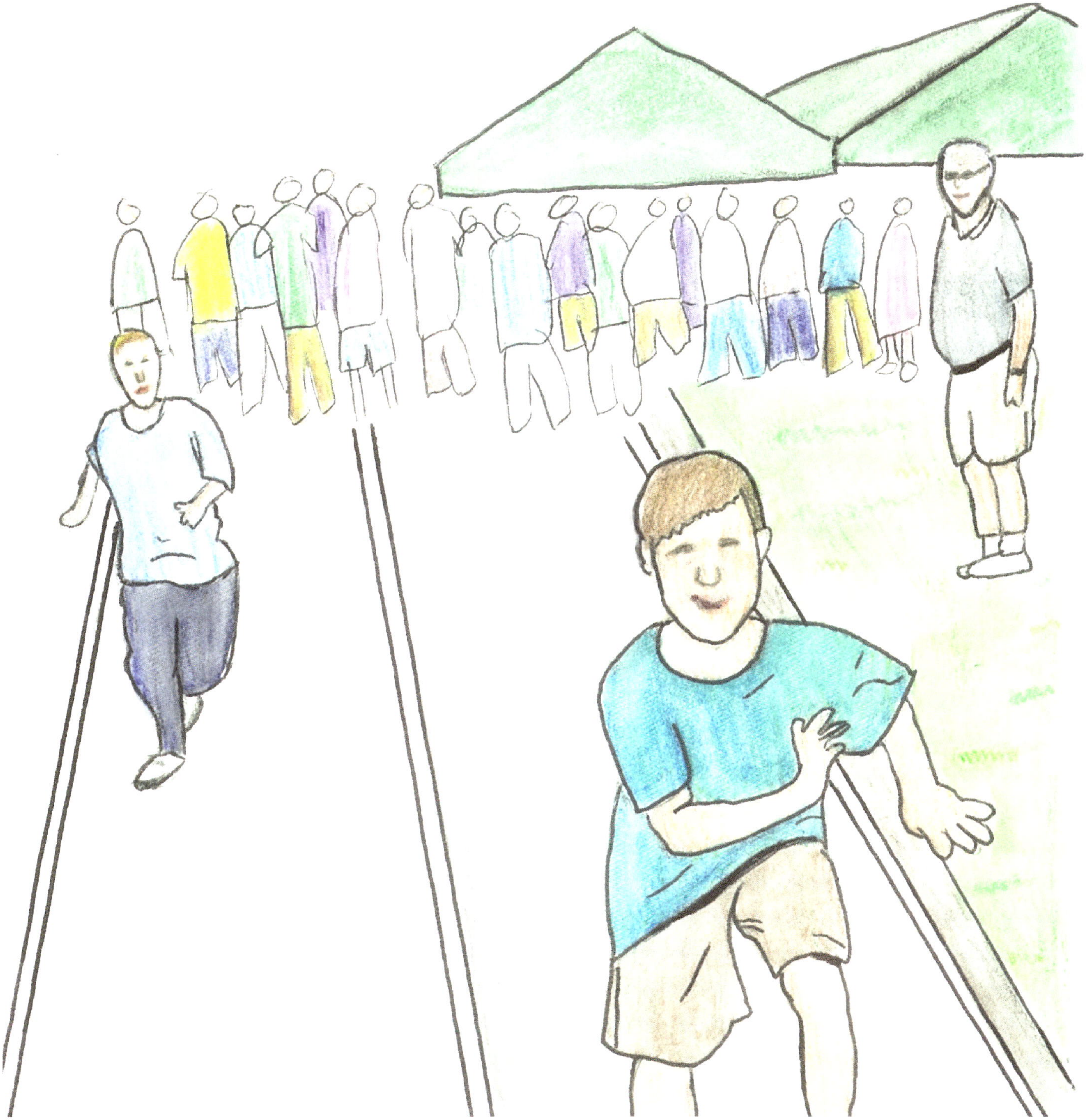

Colin doesn't worry about what anyone will think of his handwriting. It makes him happy to write thank you notes. And that makes Colin a gentleman.

COLIN INGRAHAM

Think you ate
nice piceo N [illegible]
get COLIN Nocte ga
movies for cookes
Love COLIN Nocte

Colin doesn't worry what anyone will think of his art. It makes him happy to draw. And that makes Colin an artist.

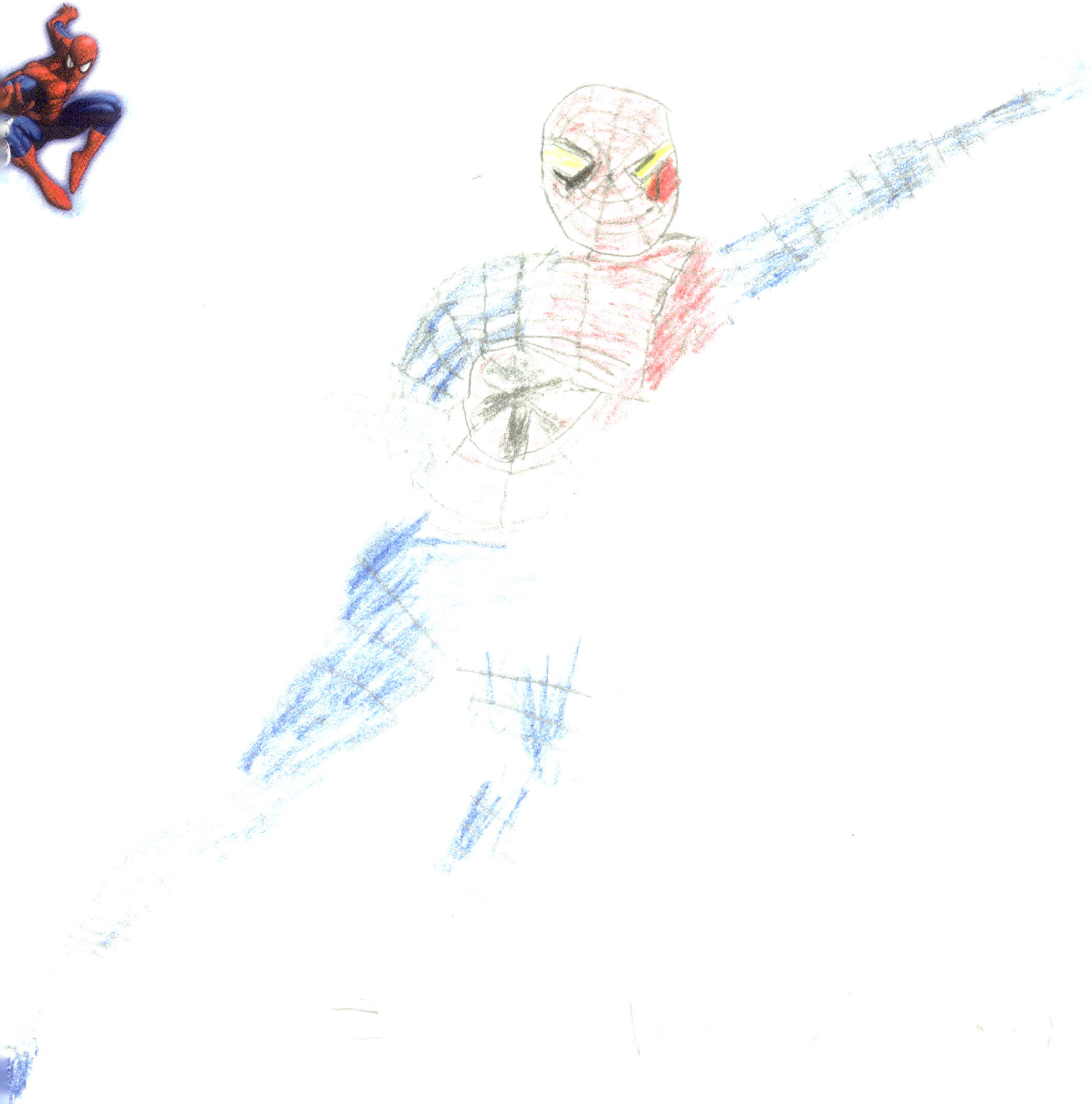

Colin talks to Jesus and that makes him a child of God.

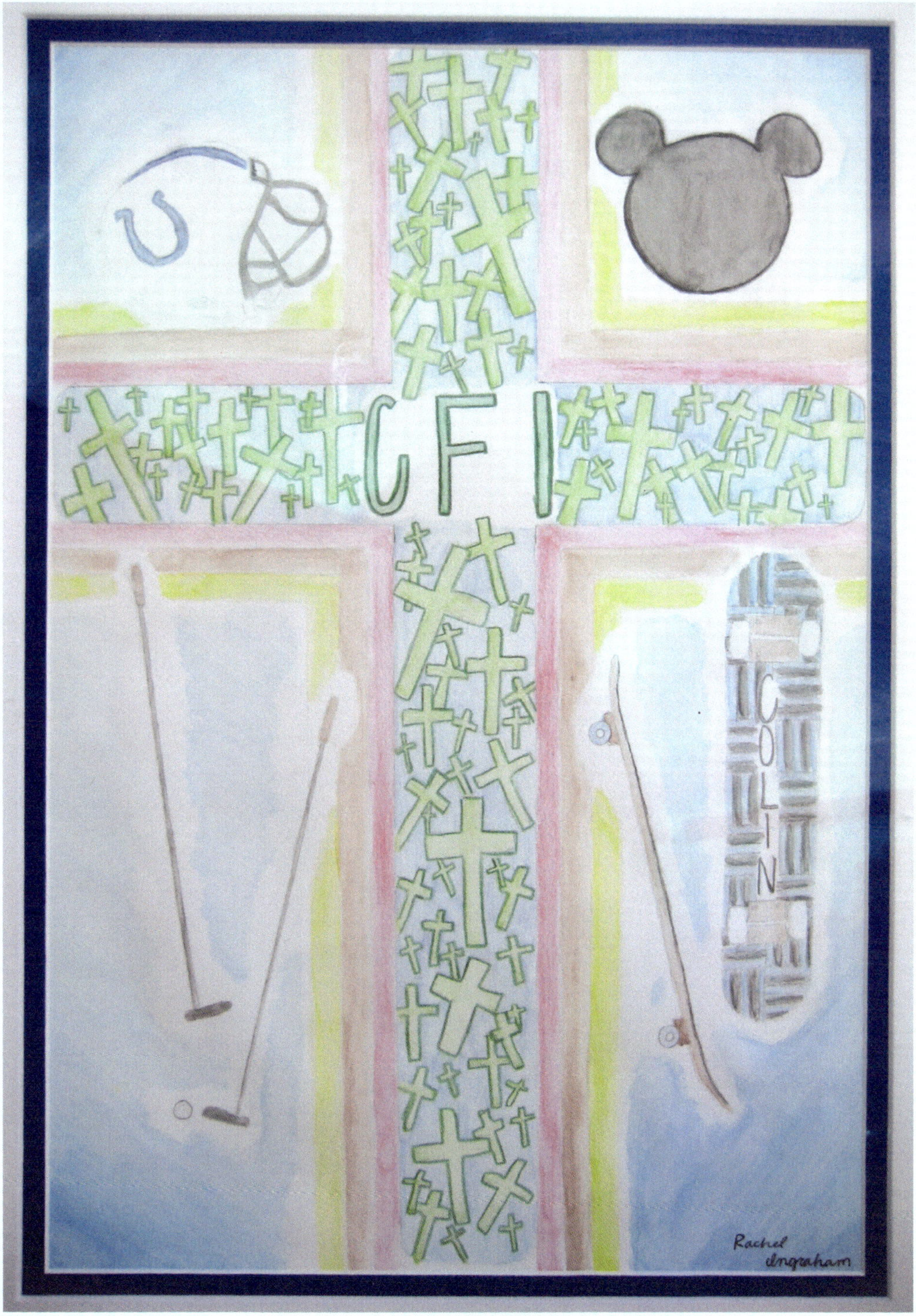
CFI
COLLIN
Rachel Ingraham

CPSIA information can be obtained
at www.ICGtesting.com
Printed in the USA
LVIC040517291111
256844LV00004B

* 9 7 8 1 4 5 6 7 3 1 0 8 3 *